IN LOVING SUPPORT
OF
SHIRLEY MAE VESTERBY COLABELLA

"DON'T COUNT THE DAYS-MAKE THE DAYS COUNT!"

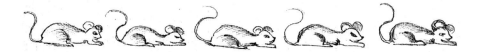

Published by
RAVENNA PRESS
2910 E. 57TH AVE. STE #10B-310
SPOKANE, WA 99223
WWW.RAVENNAPRESS.COM
"CHEMO CAT " ISBN  9780979192142
PRINTED IN THE UNITED STATES OF AMERICA
LIBRARY OF CONGRESS
CONTROL #2007926196

# Foreward to Chemo Cat by Julie R. Gralow, M.D.

Facing a new diagnosis of cancer is a challenge. Making one's way through a myriad of biopsies, scans, and surgeries, and constantly wondering what the next test will show, wreaks havoc on the patient and the entire family. A cancer diagnosis means an unpleasant disruption in our lives, being subject to painful and toxic treatments, worrying about what the future will hold, and confronting our own mortality. As medical oncologist specializing in breast cancer, it's my job to help each patient achieve the best possible survival – and that frequently includes recommending and prescribing chemotherapy, with all of its uncomfortable and much-feared side effects.

I first met Cathy Nilon at the end of 2004, shortly after her diagnosis of breast cancer at age 43. Her son, Luca, was 4 years old. Being a young mother while dealing with cancer added additional complications and issues – what should she tell her child, how would he react, would she survive to raise him? Fear was her most overwhelming emotion on that first visit - fear of a total disruption in her family's lives, fear of the toxicity of the treatment, fear of nausea and losing her hair and losing months of her life, and fear that she would not be around to watch her son grow up. She did not want to accept her cancer diagnosis, she did not want to undergo chemotherapy - she simply did not want to have to deal with any of this! But her primary goal was to do everything possible to have the best chance of being there for Luca. Gradually, with repeat visits to the cancer center, the initiation of chemotherapy, and the passing of each chemotherapy treatment, I witnessed Cathy's fear turn into courage, patience and grace. Although parts of her life were out of her control, she started taking control of the things she could. Her once negative attitude flipped to the positive. As part of her physical healing, she took up exercise to help fight her chemotherapy-related fatigue, training for and participating in a 3-day walk to raise money for breast cancer while she was still bald!

n illustrator by profession, Cathy began drawing pictures of her treatment journey as part of her
notional healing. Since her nieces' longstanding nickname for her was Cat Cat, the pictures took the
rm of a cat family. Luca joined in, supplying his thoughts and perspective on the experience. Together
ey worked to create this wonderful book, "Chemo Cat." I adore the story and the wonderful pictures
the Cat family dealing with Cat Cat's chemotherapy. Losing your hair can be traumatic, perhaps even
ore so when you are a cat and that hair loss causes you to become pink, bald, and glistening all over!
nd although I've never tried fixing macaroni and cheese on the grill, as Daddy Cat does when Cat Cat is
periencing her peak nausea, I just may have to start recommending it to my patients!

day Cathy is lovelier and both physically and emotionally healthier than ever. The experience of going
rough chemotherapy put strains on the Nilon-Volpentesta family, without a doubt. But through that
perience, and through the healing process of writing this book together, they have emerged with a
althy bond, a stronger love, and a true appreciation for each and every day. Luca and Cathy hope that
hemo Cat" can help other children and parents, as a safe place to turn to when facing a new diagnosis
cancer. I am thrilled that others will have the chance to benefit from their story.

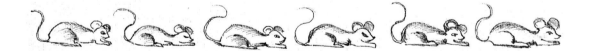

**University of Washington School of Medicine**
**Julie R. Gralow, M.D.**
**Associate Professor, Medical Oncology**
**Seattle Cancer Care Alliance**

THIS BOOK IS DEDICATED TO:

MY LOVING PARTNER BILL,

WITHOUT WHOM I HONESTLY WOULD NOT HAVE CONTINUED

TREATMENT, HE IS MY ROCK, I LOVE HIM SO MUCH;

AND TO OUR PURRRRFECT PRECIOUS LUCA

WHO GAVE ME STRENGTH, HOPE, SMILES AND LOVE.

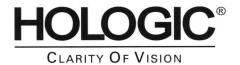

# CHEMO CAT

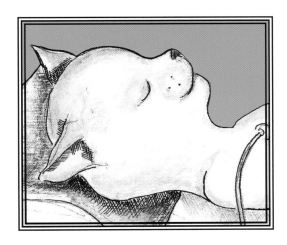

## WRITTEN & ILLUSTRATED
## BY
## CATHY NILON a.k.a. CAT- CAT
## (WITH LUCA'S HELP)

COVER DESIGN /ART DIRECTION BY KEN WHEELER
WHO SO KINDLY DONATED HIS TALENTS ON THIS PROJECT

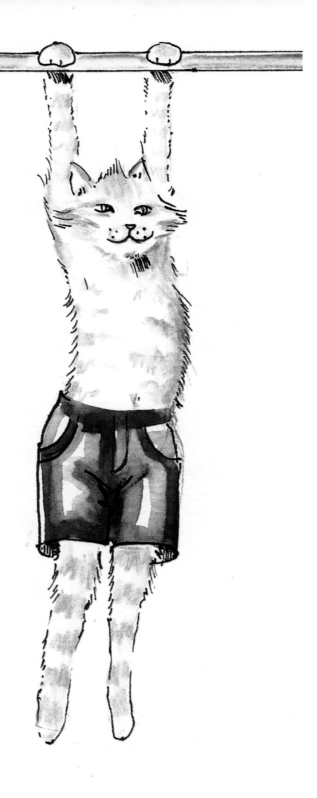

HI !

I 'M LUCA

MY MOM IS CAT-CAT
MY COUSINS KATE & ANA NAMED HER THAT

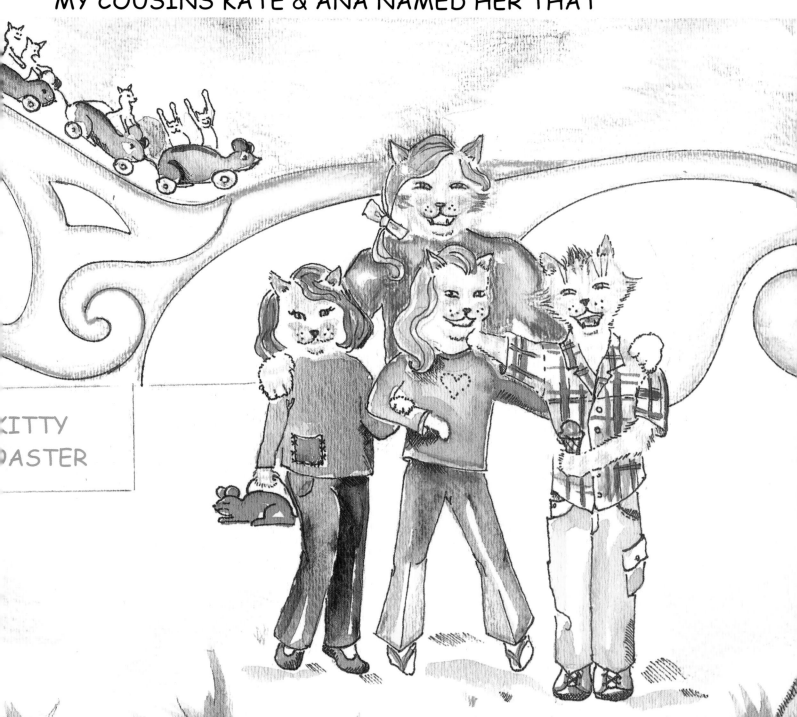

THIS IS MY DADDY-CAT BILL

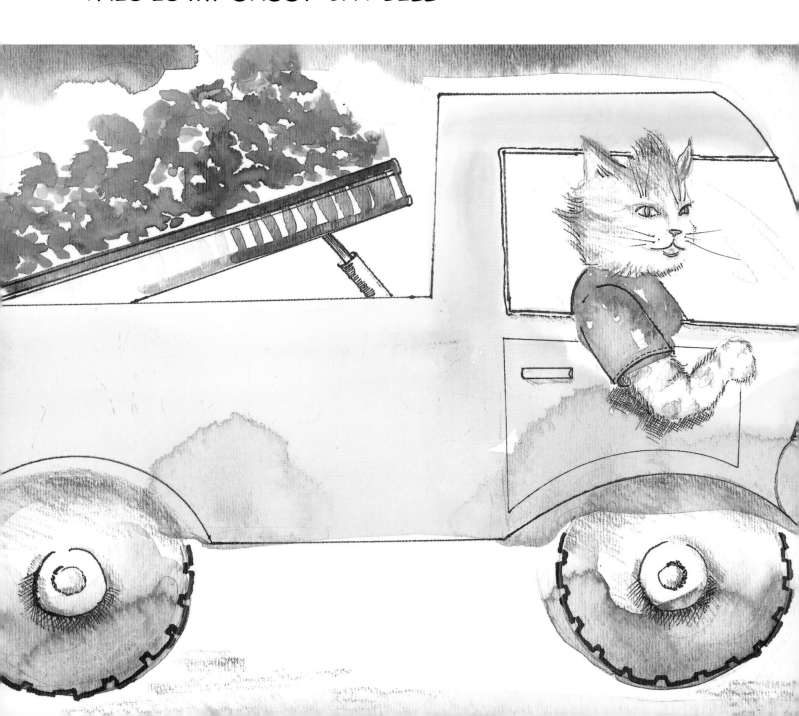

THIS STORY STARTED WHEN I WAS 4 YEARS OLD
AND CONTINUES STILL

WE ARE THE HAPPIEST FAMILY
WE LOVE TO RUN
JUMP AND PLAY

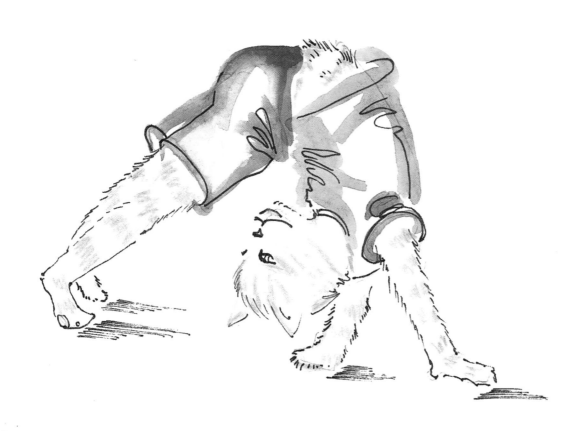

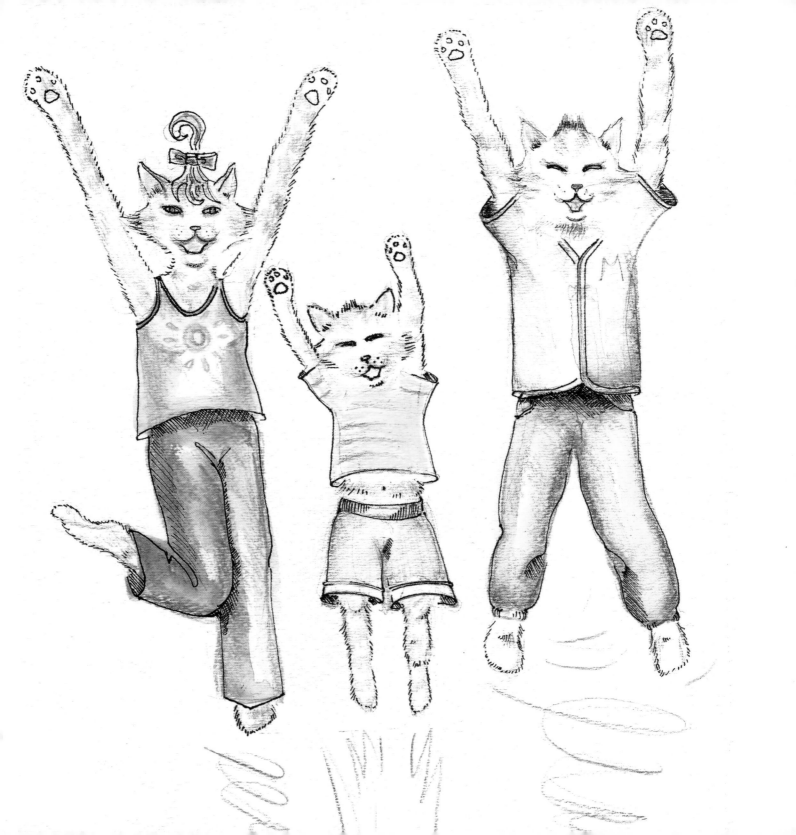

BUT ONE DIFFICULT DAY...
CAT-CAT'S DOCTOR AND HER FANCY MACHINE
FOUND A LUMP

SHE SAID IT HAD TO GO
SOMETHING CALLED CHEMO
WOULD BE NEEDED
TO KILL THIS CANCER  BUMP

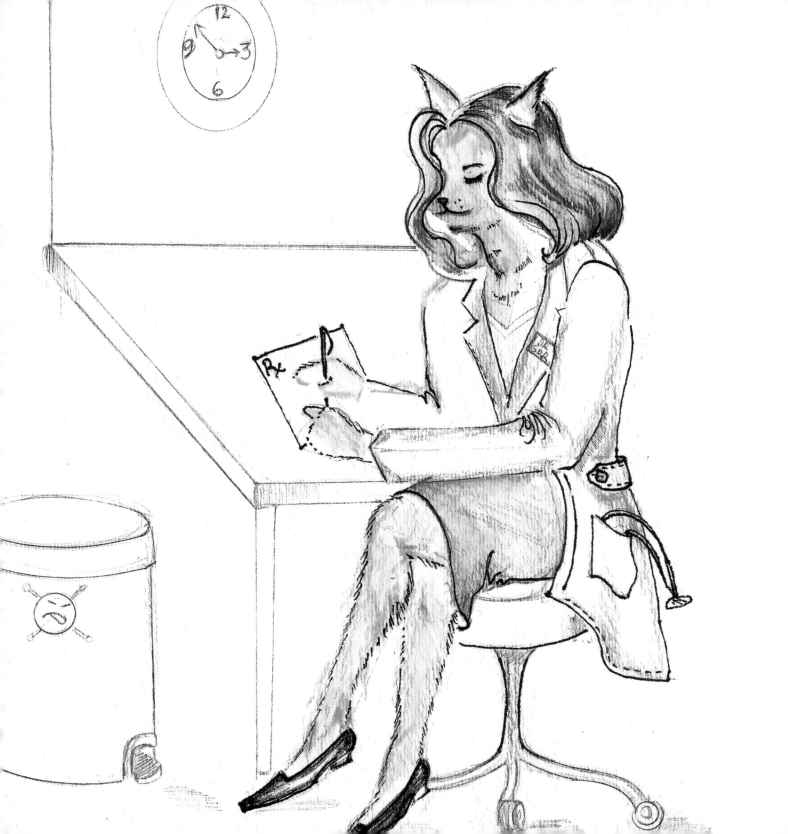

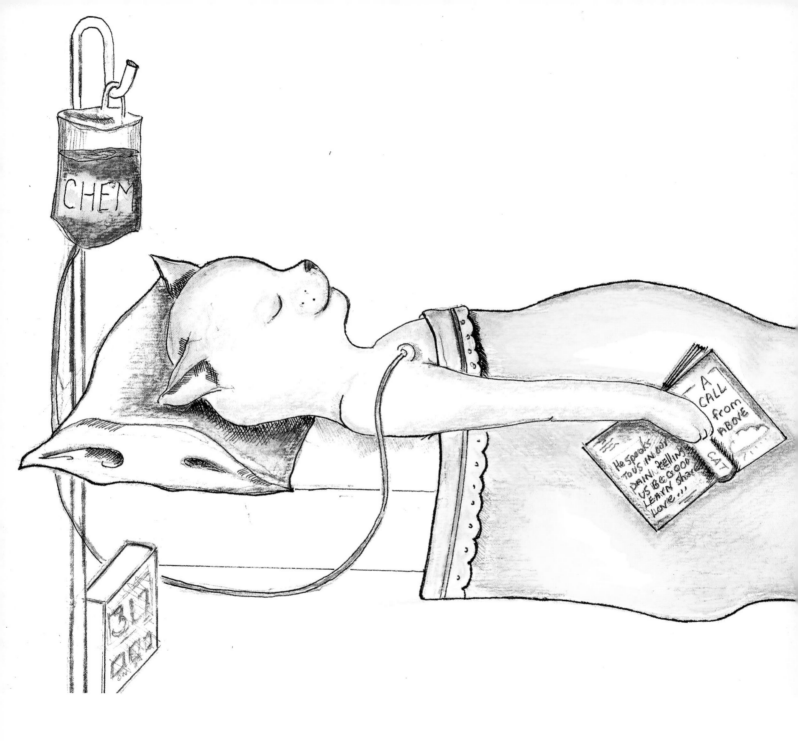

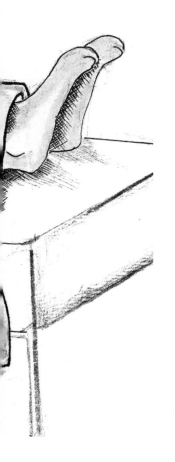

IT WOULD TAKE TIME
BEFORE SHE WOULD BE FINE

THINGS WOULD BE DIFFERENT FOR A WHILE
THERE WOULD BE CHANGES
IN OUR LIFE STYLE

CAT-CAT WAS TOLD THERE'D BE
PROBLEMS FROM THE MEDICINE SHE TOOK...

ONE WAS THAT HER HAIR ...

WOULD FALL OUT WHILE SHE LOOKED!

IT WOULD SLOWLY COME OUT
   IT WOULD FALL ON THE FLOOR
      AND THEN IT WOULD SIMPLY
              BE NO MORE...


SHE WOULD BE PINK, BALD AND GLISTENING
LIKE A NEWBORN BABY PIG

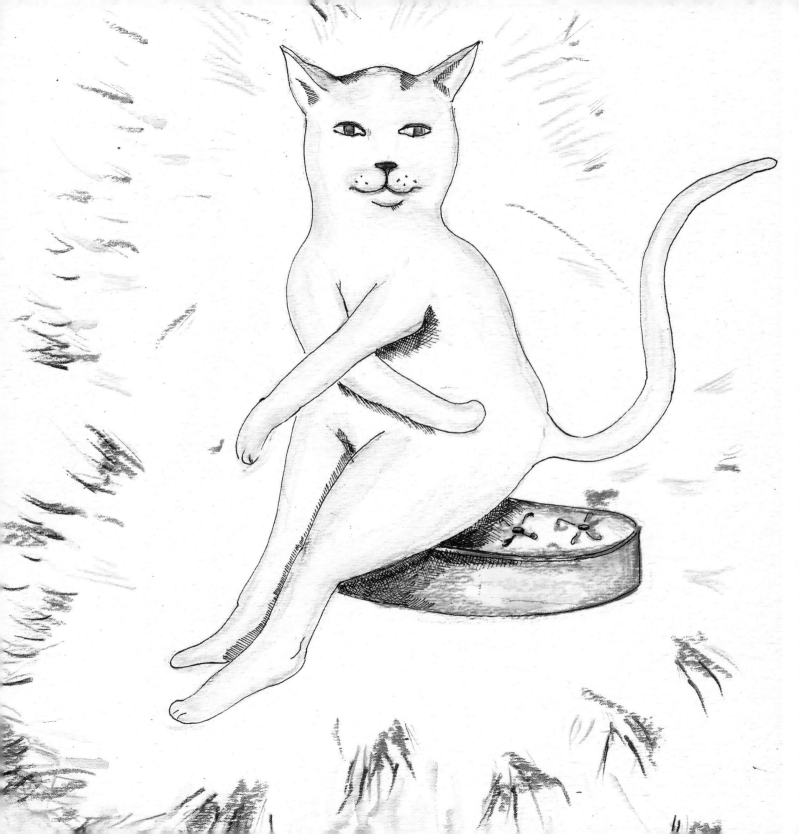

SO...THE COUSINS
CAME WITH US
TO THE WIG SHOP

WE HELPED CAT- CAT
TRY ON
AND PICK OUT....

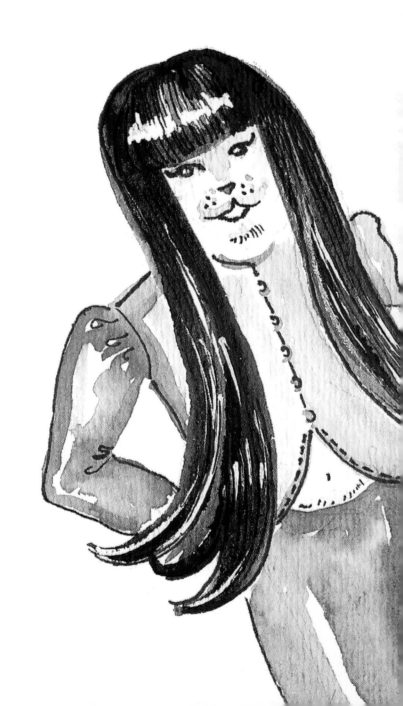

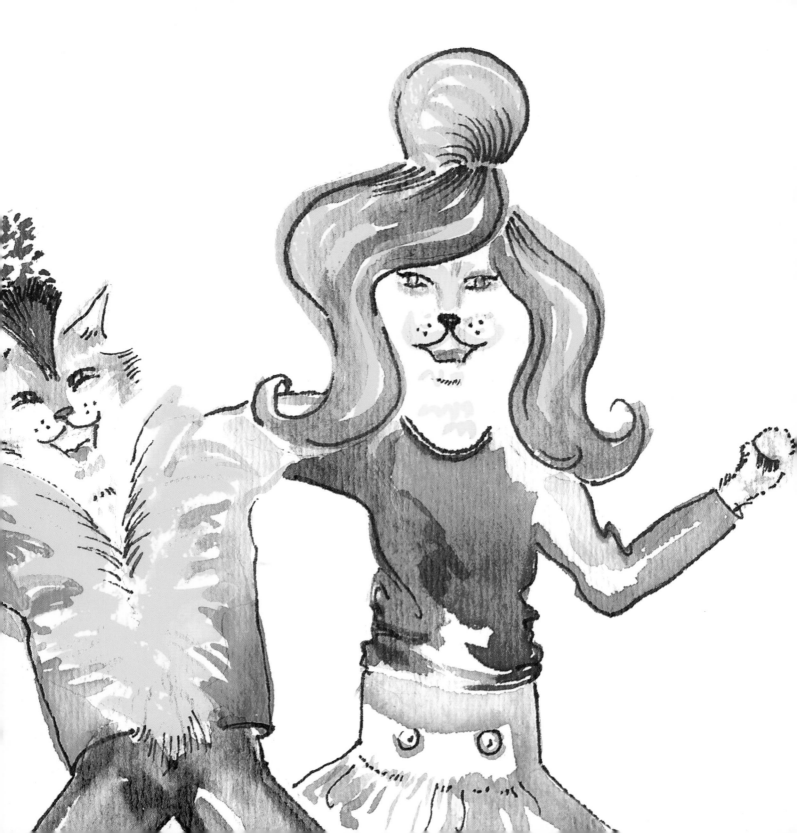

# ...SOME NEW GOLDEN LOCKS

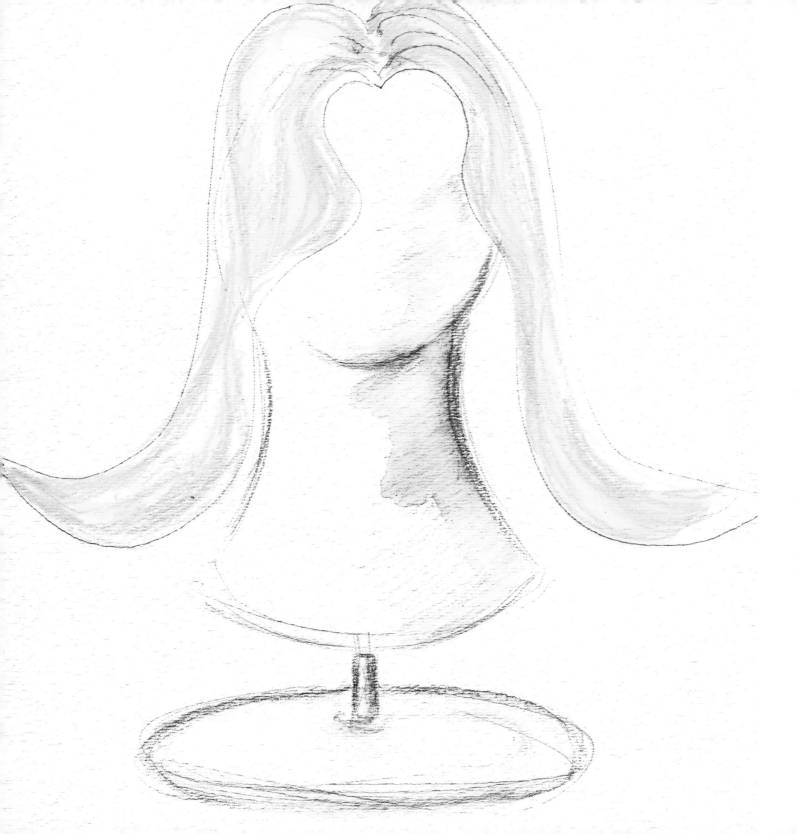

MY JOB WAS TO PLAY CHESS
CHECKERS AND BINGO
SO NOT TO MAKE NOISE

NO BOUNCING ON THE BED OR
PLAYING WITH LOUD TOYS

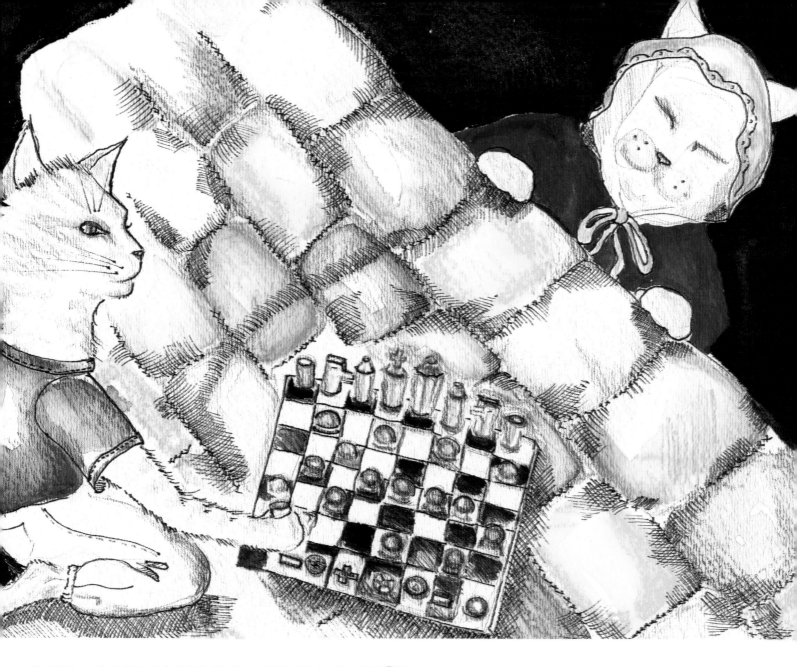

CAT- CAT SHOULD STAY QUIET
AND GET LOTS OF REST
TO STOP THE CANCER THAT GREW IN HER BREAST

DADDY CAT MADE THE MOST
KITTY-LICIOUS MEALS...
LIKE MAC AND CHEESE ON THE GRILL

THIS HELPED CAT-CAT'S STOMACH
BETTER THAN PILLS

HE WORKED HARD
NOT TO SHOW HIS FEAR
HE WORRIED ABOUT CAT- CAT
WHOM HE LOVES SO DEAR

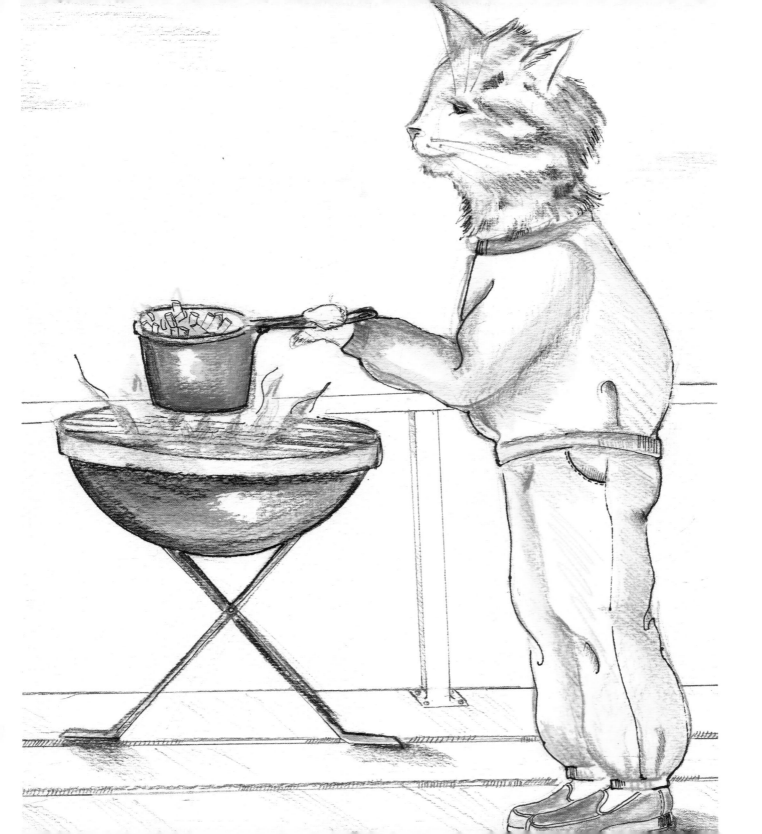

I'D BRING HER CRACKERS
ALL ORANGE AND FINE

WHICH HELPED HER TO SMILE
MOST OF THE TIME

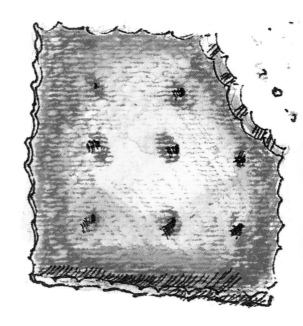

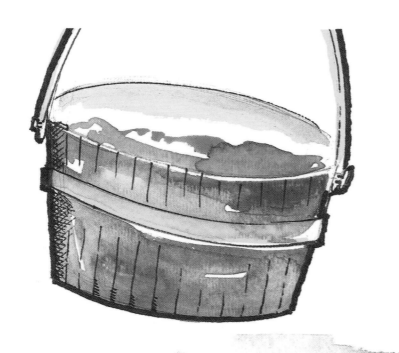

(WE KEPT THE BUCKET
NEAR TO HER BED
JUST IN CASE
SHE HAD TO THROW UP
ALL OVER THE PLACE)

SHE LOVES ME
MORE THAN THE
EARTH
SUN
AND STARS

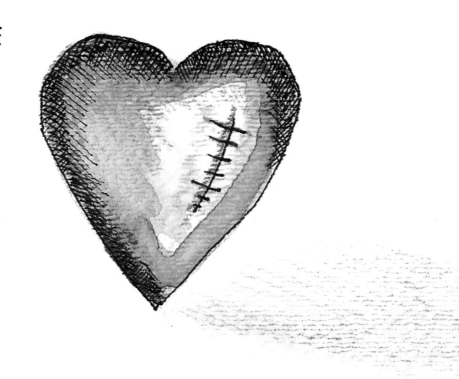

BUT CANCER IS HARD ON US
WE ALL WOULD HAVE SOME SCARS

I THINK I WAS SADDEST BY FAR
AND SOMETIMES WOULD SHOUT

OR JUST SIT ON THE FLOOR
AND CRY MY EYES OUT

I WAS TIRED OF KIDS
WHO HAD
HEALTHIER MOMS

I WISHED FOR THE DAY
I COULD RUN INTO HER ARMS...
AND HAVE PIGGY-BACK RIDES
WITHOUT DOING HER ANY HARM

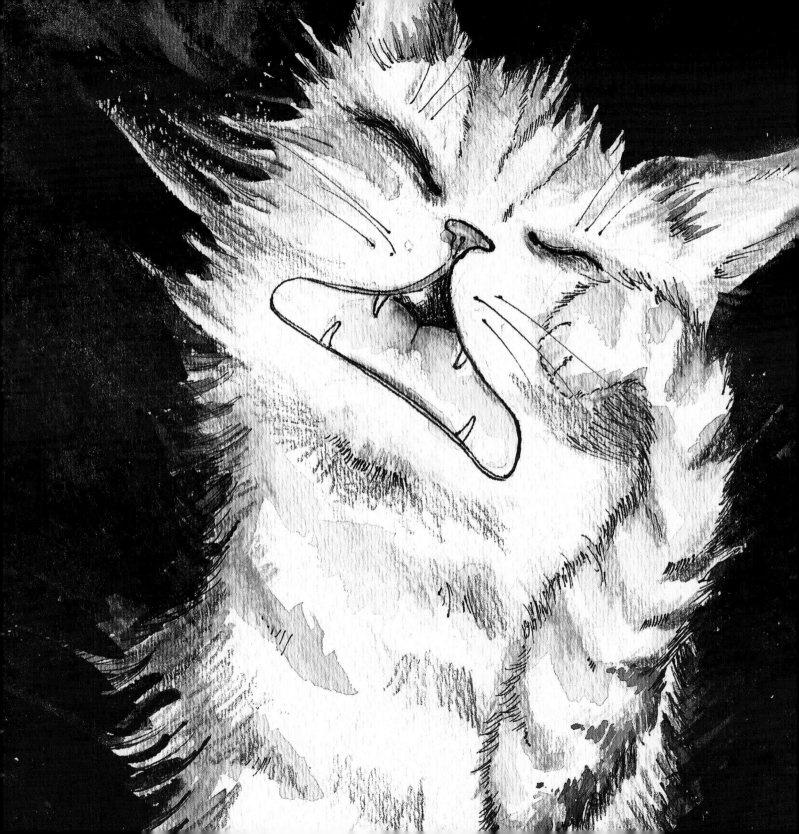

WHERE HAD HER
CANCER COME FROM?
I WISH SOMEONE KNEW!
I SECRETLY WORRIED
COULD I CATCH IT TOO?

DID IT GROW LIKE A WEED
FROM UNDER THE DECK
OR
HIDE IN THE SCARF
SHE WORE ON HER NECK?

BUT NO !
WE WERE TOLD
CANCER IS NOT CAUGHT LIKE A COLD
IT IS SOMETHING MYSTERIOUS
THAT GROWS LIKE A MOLD...

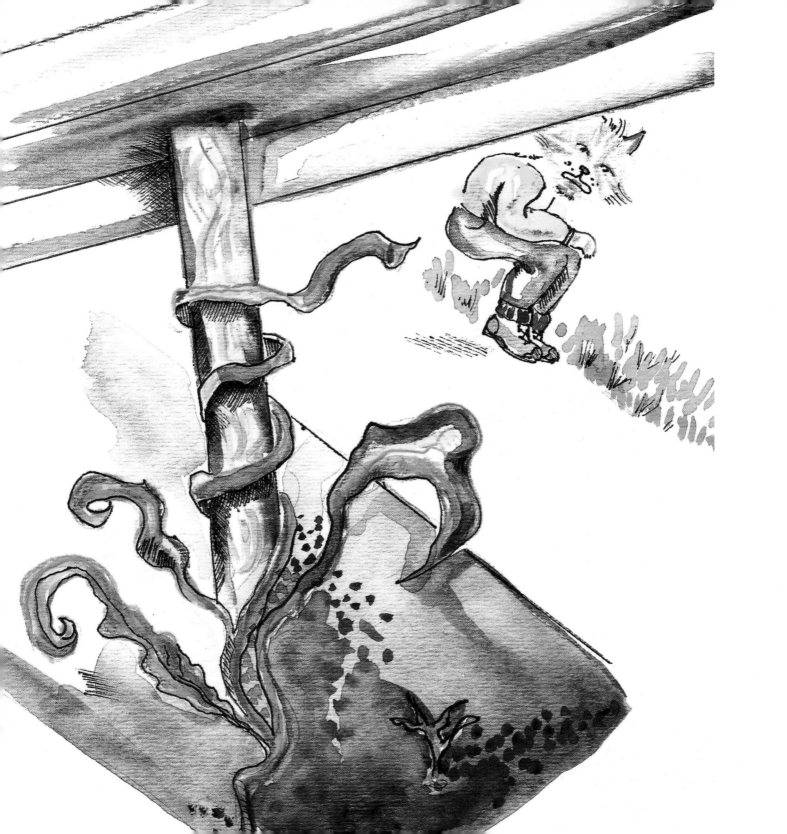

I DID NOT WANT
TO GO ALONE
TO MY PRE-SCHOOL

SO CAT-CAT CAME IN
EVERY DAY FOR A WHILE
WHICH MADE ME SMILE

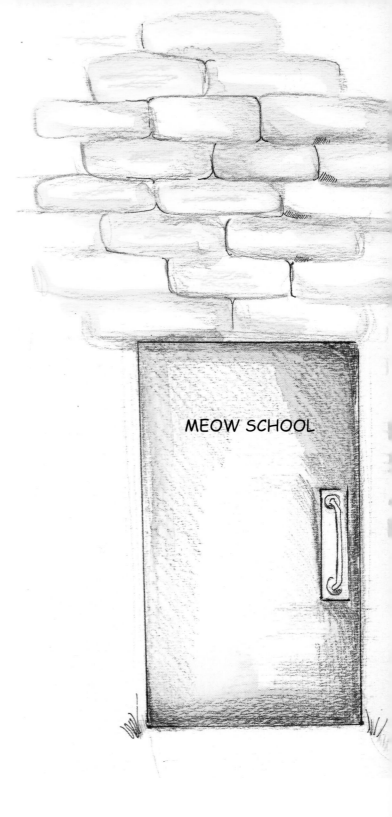

MEOW SCHOOL

SHE FELT LIKE A MESS
BUT
PUT ON HER BEST DRESS

I TOLD HER SHE LOOKED
PRETTY
HUGGED AND KISSED
HER A LOT

THIS MADE HER GET
BETTER
MUCH FASTER
THE THOUGHT

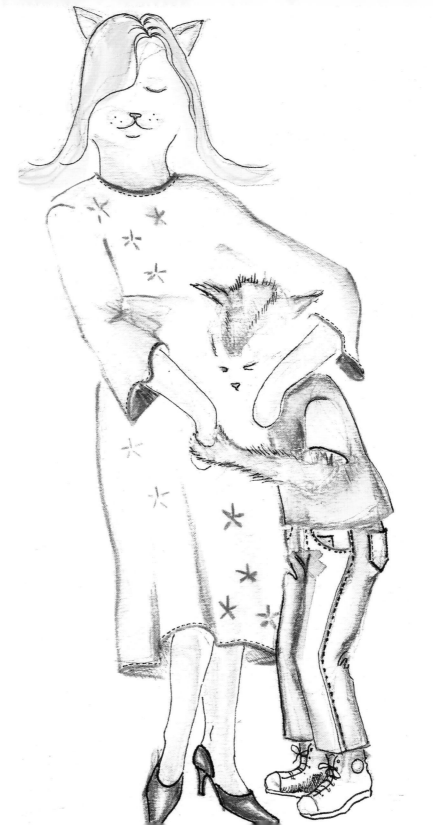

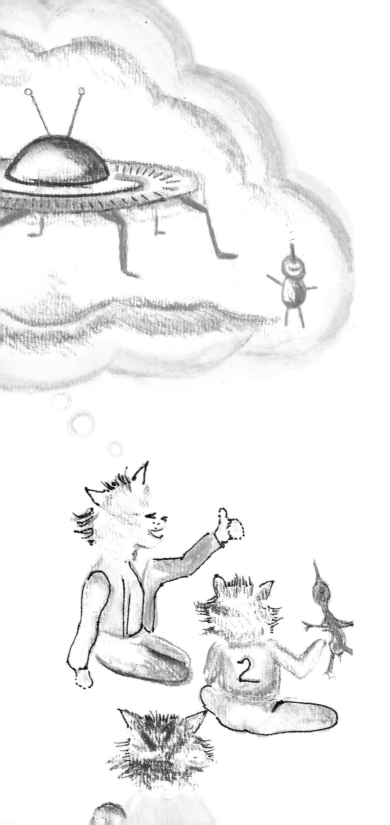

THE BOYS SAID MY MOM
LOOKED REAL COOL...

LIKE AN ALIEN THAT CAME
FROM THE MOON...

BUT
THE GIRLS TOOK ONE LOOK
AND RAN FROM THE ROOM!

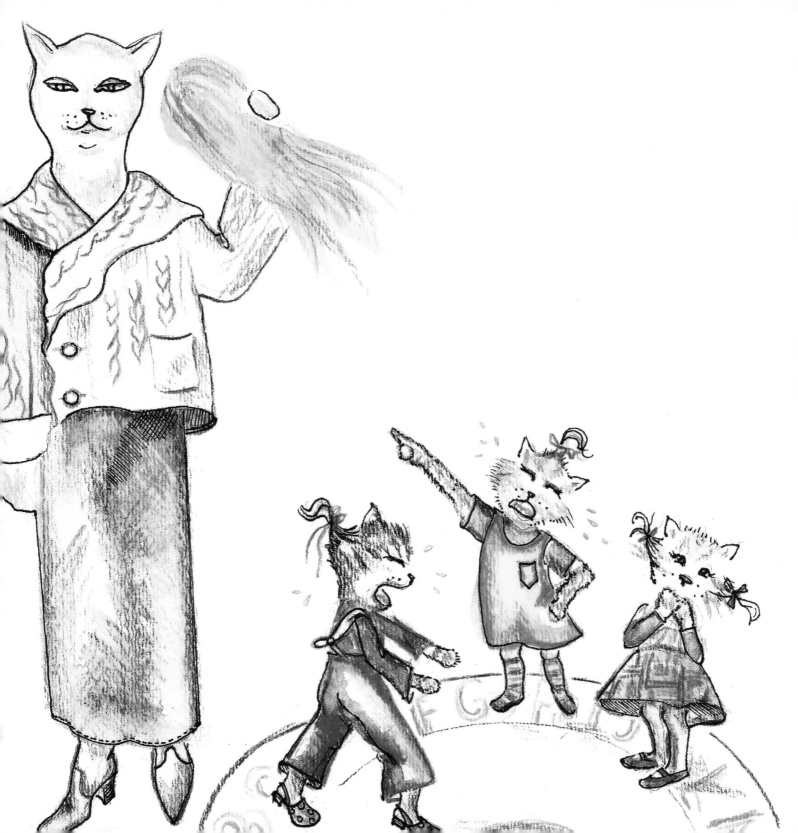

MOST DAYS CAT-CAT WOULD SLEEP IN HER ROOM
WHILE DADDY AND I TRIED TO VACUUM THE GLOOM

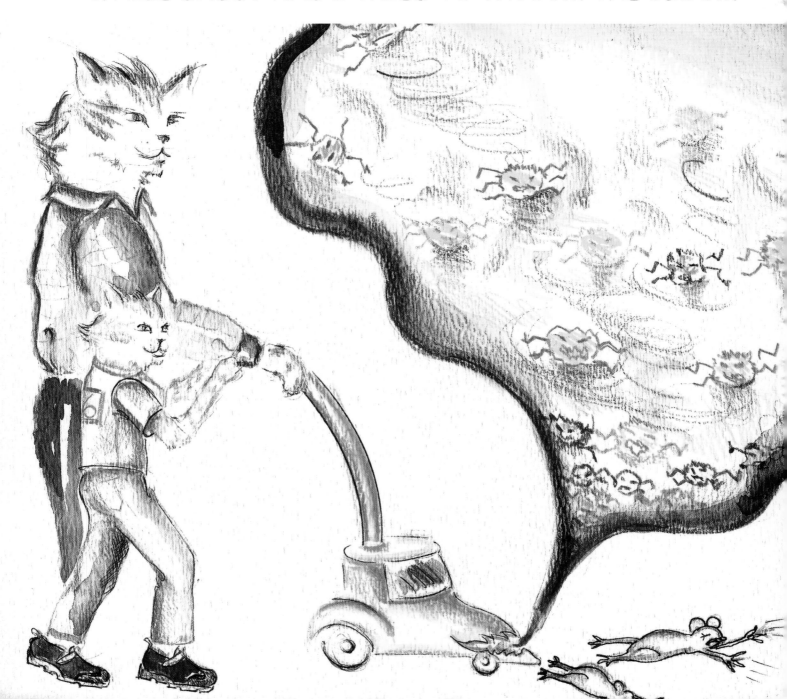

NE NIGHT
ASKED
 I'D BE GETTING
NEW MOM
HIS SPRING

HE KISSED ME
ND TOLD ME
OT TO THINK
UCH A THING

HE WOULD
LWAYS
 MY MAMA
 MATTER
HAT LIFE
OULD BRING

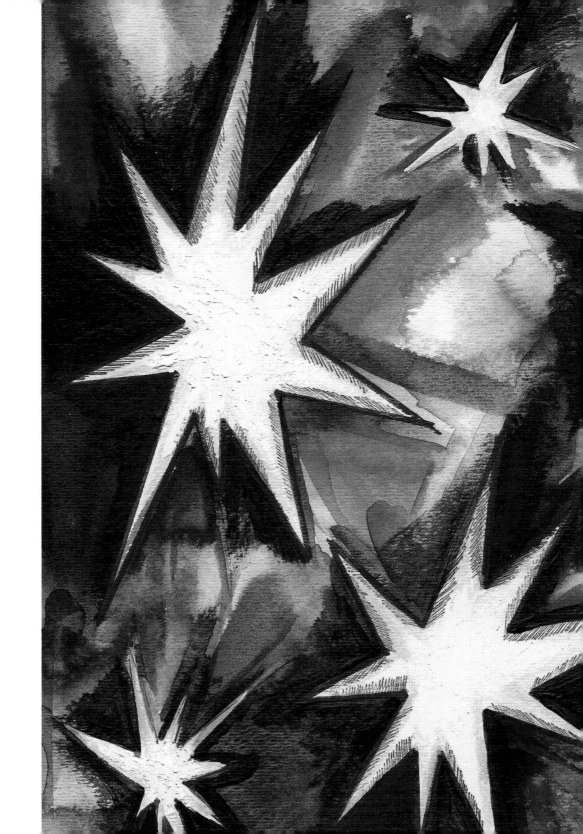

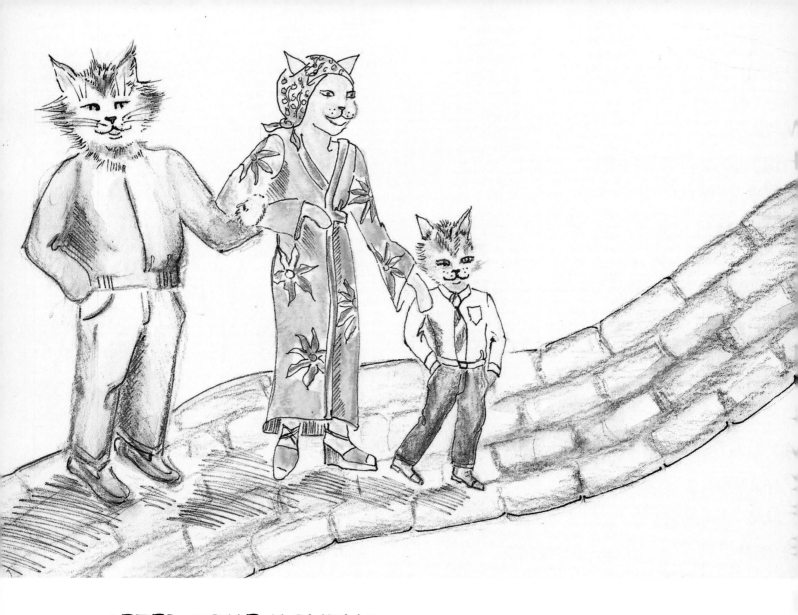

AFTER SOME MONTHS
THE CHEMO WAS OVER
AND CAT-CAT FINALLY STARTED TO FEEL BETTER...

WE DECIDED TO SEND OUT
HUNDREDS OF LETTERS
TO GET FUNDS AND SUPPORT
TO HELP LOTS OF OTHERS

CAT-CAT WALKED TO RAISE MONEY
WITH FRIENDS
DADS AND MOTHERS

HOPING THE DOCTORS COULD FIND
A CURE
CAUSE OR ANSWER
FOR THIS DIFFICULT
BREAST CANCER

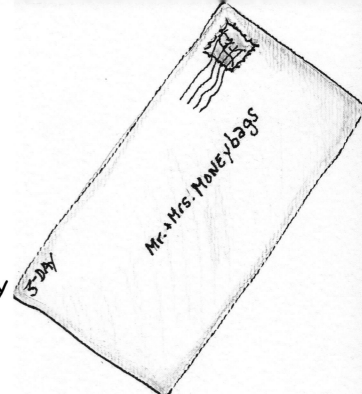

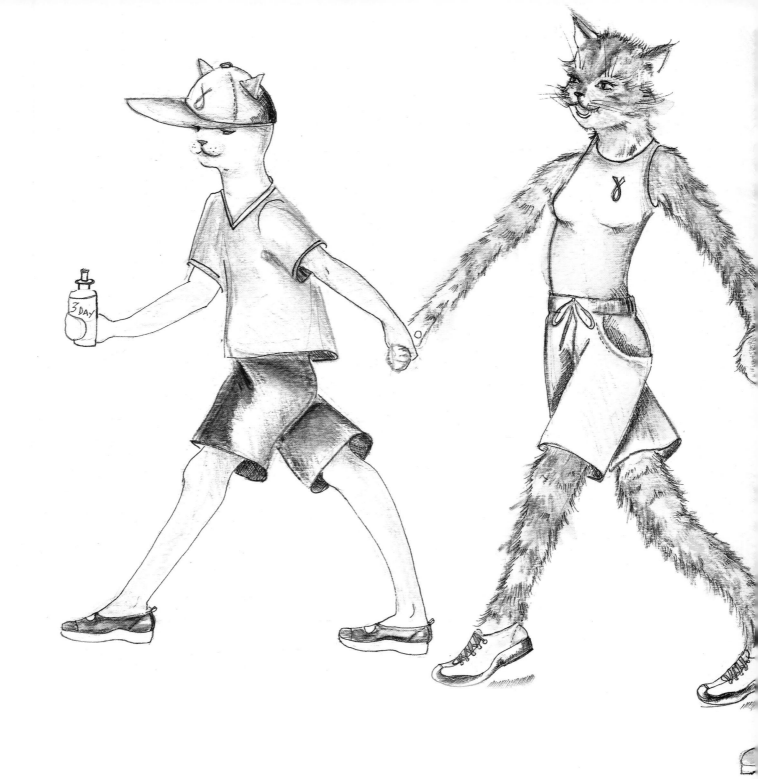

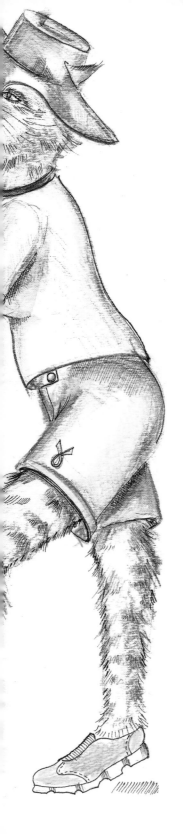

HER FRIENDS HAD PROVEN
THEY WERE THERE TO STAY

NOW SHE HELD THEIR HANDS
LEADING THE WAY

AS THEY WALKED AND WALKED
THAT BRIGHT SUNNY DAY

CAT-CAT'S HAIR CAME BACK
A GROOVY NEW COLOR...

IT WAS DIFFERENT BY FAR
THAN THE HAIR IN THE JAR

WE HAD  PICKED UP
FROM THE FLOOR
JUST ONE YEAR  BEFORE

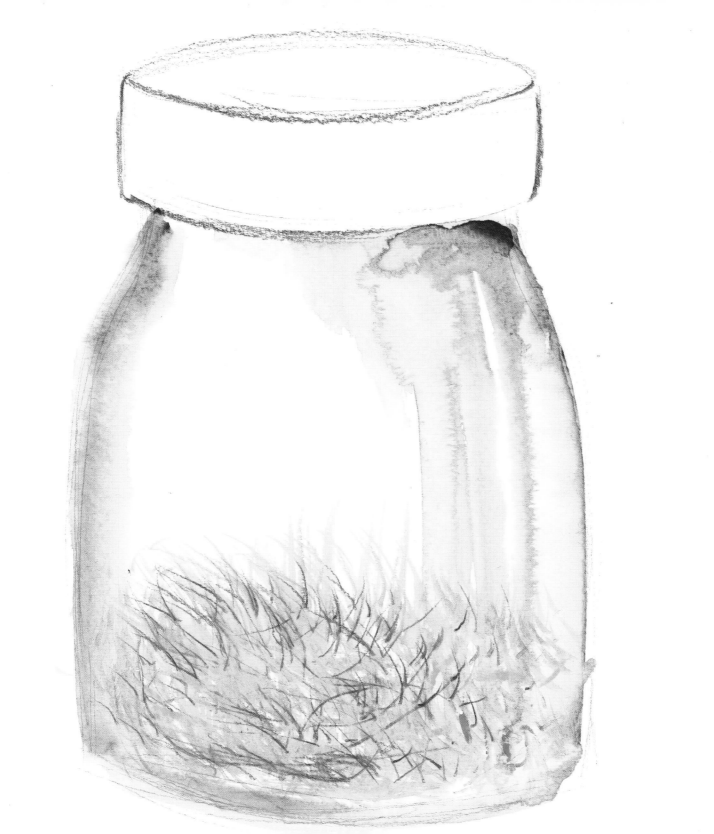

WE WENT TO THE BEACH
AND SAT ON THE SAND
I REACHED OVER TO HOLD
MAMA'S THIN HAND
I KISSED HER SO GENTLY
ALL OVER HER FACE

THIS HAD BEEN A ROUGH YEAR ...
TEACHING COURAGE
PATIENCE AND
GRACE

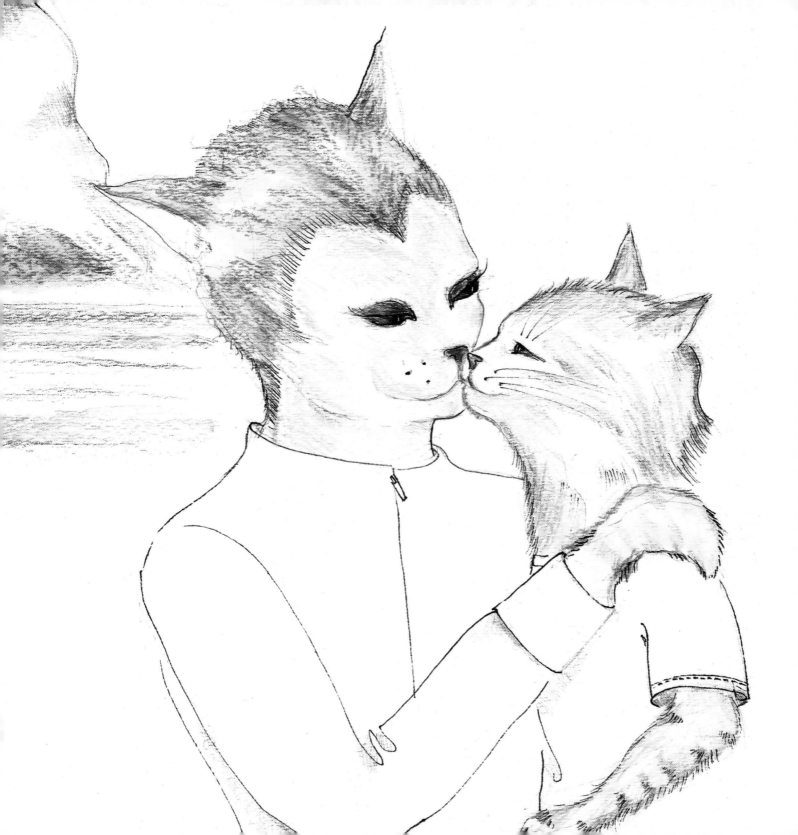

AT SCHOOL WE MET
ANOTHER YOUNG MOTHER
WHO HAD JUST BEGUN
THE VERY SAME FIGHT
I ASKED CAT- CAT IF SHE
WOULD BE ALRIGHT?

MAMA SAID WITH OUR HELP
MANY BLESSINGS AND CAKE
SHE WOULD HOPEFULLY
LIVE TO 108

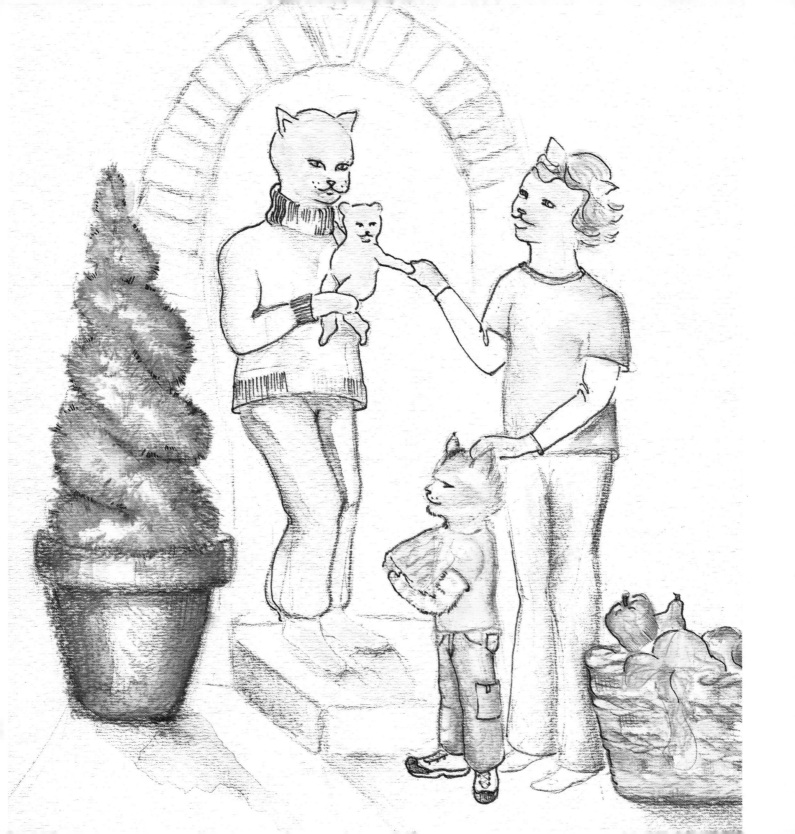

I WANTED TO FINISH THIS LITTLE BOOK
TO GIVE OTHER FAMILIES A GOOD PLACE TO LOOK
TO SEE THAT THEY'LL BE OK !
WITH STRENGTH AND LOVE
THEY'LL GET THROUGH EACH DAY
AND
WITH FAITH
FRIENDS AND FAMILY
WE ALL FIND THE WAY

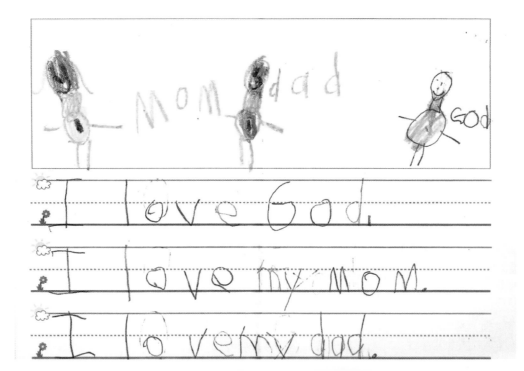

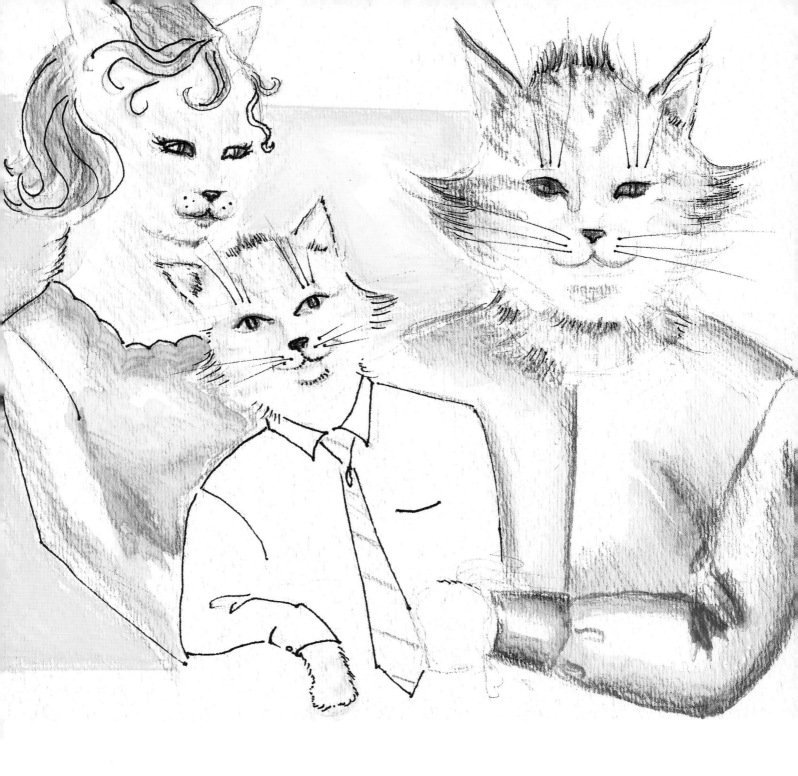

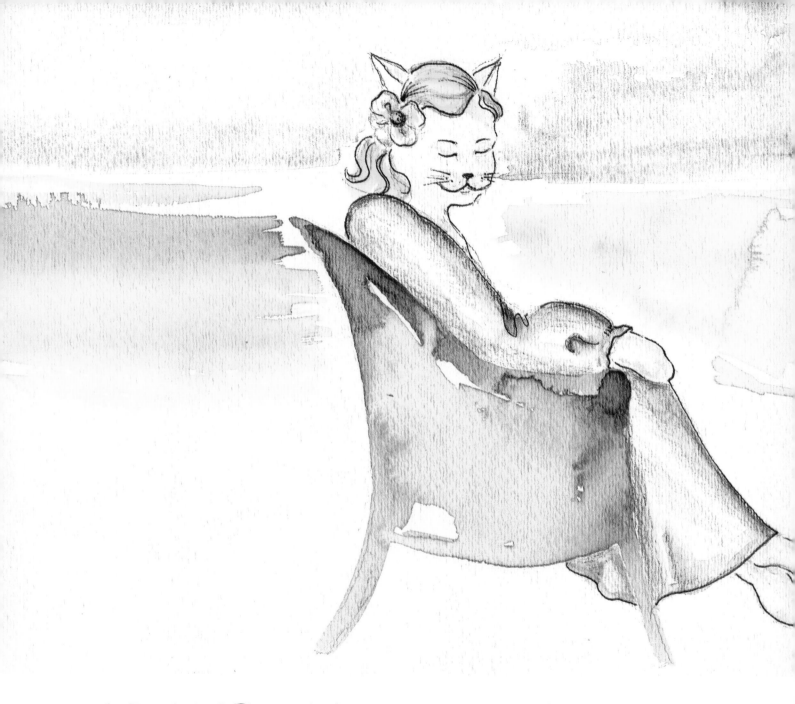

CAT- CAT RELAXING IN HAWAII ONE YEAR
AFTER CHEMO ENDS

# A NEW BEGINNING....

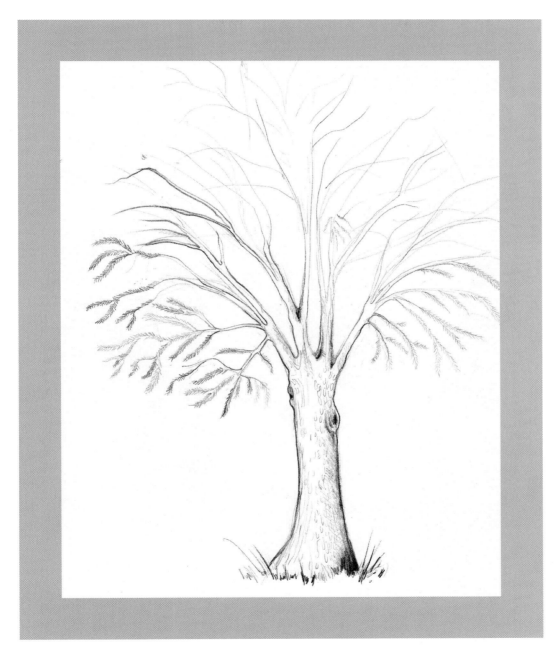

NEVER ....."THE END"

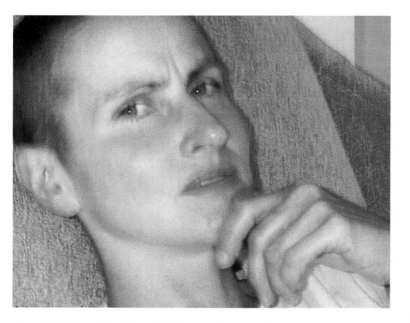

CATHY AFTER 2ND A/C CHEMO
TREATMENT (LOOKING DAZED AND
CONFUSED)

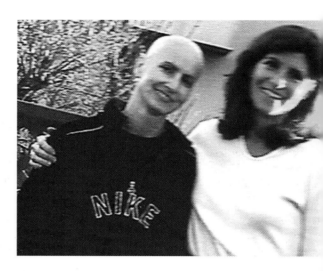

CATHY WITH BEST FRIEND ANN
WHO HELPED DAILY-ALONG WIT
HER SWEET SON MATT

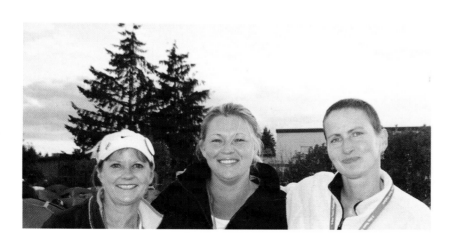

JUDY, COLLEEN AND CATHY
3 DAY WALK

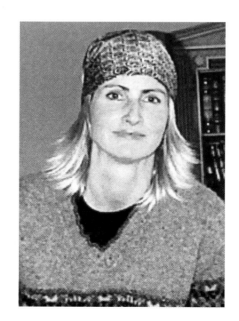

WIG TIED WITH GRANDMA'S
SILK SCARF

Chemo Cat's author and illustrator Cathy Nilon is a native New Yorker now living with her life partner Bill and their son Luca in the Seattle, WA area.

Cathy plans to continue writing and illustrating books with uplifting themes for children of all ages.  She is a lifelong cat lover and currently Gracie and Piggy complete their very grateful family.

Educated in New York City at the High School of Art and Design and the Fashion Institute of Technology, as well as Ars Sutoria in Milan, Italy, the internationally acclaimed school for shoe design, she has had an extensive career in shoe design and production most recently for Liz Claiborne  living for long periods of time in Italy, Indonesia, Taiwan, China and Hong Kong.  She has come full circle back to her early dreams of writing and illustrating children's books.

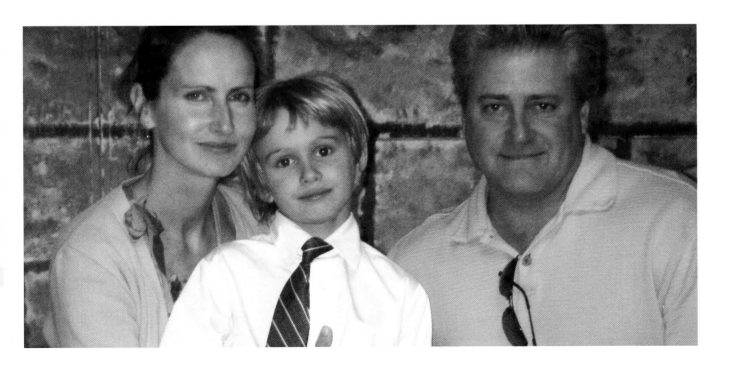

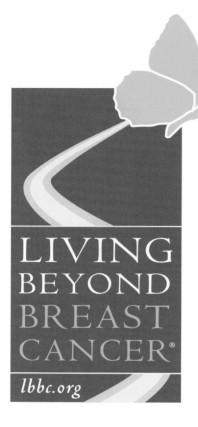

The Author's net proceeds will be donated to:

Living Beyond Breast Cancer, founded in 1991, a national nonprofit education and support organizatio dedicated to empowering all women affected by breast cancer to live as long as possible with the best quality of life. Programs and services include: large-scale interactive conferences; teleconferences; the Survivors' Helpline (888.753.5222), a toll-free information and support line; www.lbbc.org, an informational website; free quarterly newsletters; publications for medically underserved women, including young women, women with advanced (metastatic) breast cancer and women of color; low-cost informational recordings; networking programs; workshops and trainings for healthcare providers; and the Paula A. Seidman Library and Resource Center.

A Note From Cathy;

So many generous and loving souls came to help my family during this crisis.
When I tried to list all of those people that I wanted to personally thank
and acknowledge ...it became another short story.
Those people know who they are, angels on earth.
I will never forget each act of kindness as long as I live.
Thank you for teaching me to receive. I encourage all people reading this
to reach out to those in need.  My prayers of healing go out to the many
families  who have lost loved ones to cancer.  Email: chemocat@gmail.com

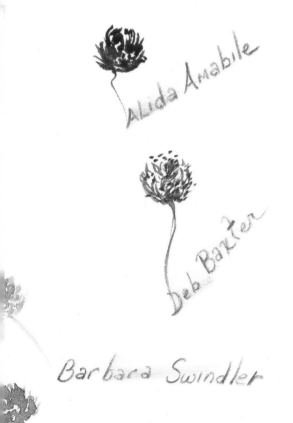

Alida Amabile

Deb Baxter

Barbara Swindler

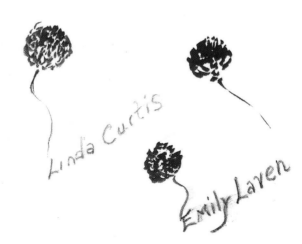

Linda Curtis

Emily Laven

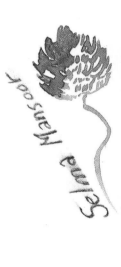

Selma Mansoor